Pocke ||||||||||||||||||||||||||||||||

Cancer

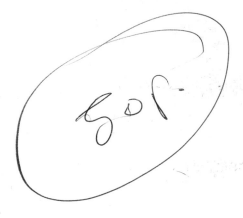

An **Essential Slide Collection of Cancer**, based on the contents of this book, is available. The collection consists of numbered 35mm colour transparencies of each illustration in the book. The material is presented in an attractive binder, which also contains a copy of the Pocket Picture Guide. The Essential Slide Collection is available from:

Mosby Europe Limited
Brook House
2–16 Torrington Place
London WC1E 7LT
UK

Pocket Picture Guides

Cancer

Dr Jeffrey S Tobias
MA (Cantab), MD, FRCP, FRCR
Clinical Director
Department of Clinical Oncology
University College and Middlesex Hospitals
London

Dr Christopher J Williams
DM, FRCP
Senior Lecturer in Medical Oncology and
Honorary Consultant Physician
University of Southampton
Southampton General Hospital
Southampton

ᴍWOLFE

London St. Louis Baltimore Boston Chicago Philadelphia Sydney Toronto

British Library Cataloguing in Publication Data:
available on request

Library of Congress Cataloging in Publication Data:
available on request

ISBN 1-57375-616-1

Publisher:	Fiona Foley
Project Manager:	Moira Sarsfield
Design:	James Evoy
Index:	Anne McCarthy
Production:	Susan Bishop

Printed and originated in Hong Kong
Produced by Mandarin Offset (Hong Kong) Ltd

Preface

Cancer remains a vast medical problem with a high mortality. Both in the United States and in Europe, efforts to reduce cancer deaths by the year 2000 have attracted major government support and funding, yet the present methods of treatment still lack precision, and in many cases our best efforts at cure or long-term control remain unsuccessful. On the other hand, the past decade has seen a dramatic increase in our understanding of biological mechanisms, of the importance of neoplastic cell growth and in the potential of cytokines and other growth factors both in the development of cancer and perhaps in the future as a further means of treatment.

This little volume provides an illustrated overview of some of the more common and visible effects of cancer, for non-specialists who are interested in the subject as well as trainee and practising oncologists and physicians in related specialities. We hope that the book may also be of interest to medical students who wish to know more about this critically important but often neglected part of their studies. We have attempted to provide typical examples of some of the more serious problems most frequently encountered in normal clinical practice, though therapy, evaluation and prognosis are largely outside the scope of this book.

For the clinician, management of the common cancers and of the complications of their treatment provides a fascinating and varied series of challenges. We hope that the illustrations in this small volume will give the reader both an insight into some of these problems and a renewed interest in exploring further the needs of the cancer patient.

Contents

Clinical Behaviour

Cancers are characterized by uncontrolled cell division of a malignant clone, generally from a single primary site.

A common (but not invariable) feature of many cancers is metastatic spread with wide dissemination. An understanding of the metastatic behaviour of different tumour types is very important in planning the management of the disease.

The main routes of spread in human tumours are by direct local extension, lymphatic involvement, and haematogenous metastases. Some brain tumours seed only into the cerebrospinal fluid, and extensive spread within the abdominal cavity (trans-coelemic spread) is particularly characteristic of ovarian cancer.

CLONALITY OF TUMOURS

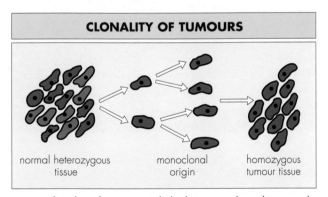

normal heterozygous tissue

monoclonal origin

homozygous tumour tissue

Fig. 1 Clonality of tumours. X-linked enzymes have been used to study this feature of tumours. One such study looked at the two isoenzymes of glucose-6-phosphate dehydrogenase in heterozygous black females. Although normal tissue produced both isoenzymes, tumour tissue was found to express only one or the other. This observation is consistent with the hypothesis that the tumour tissue arose from a single cell.

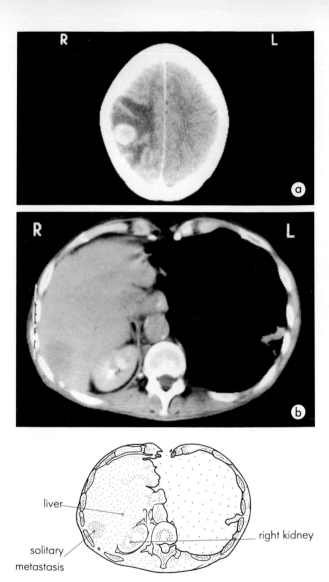

Fig. 2 Late systemic relapse. This may occur many years after initial diagnosis and surgery in cancers associated with very rapid and widespread haematogenous dissemination. This implies that metastatic cells, not recognised at initial diagnosis, have the potential to remain dormant for decades. (a) Single cortical metastasis from breast cancer, 5 years after mastectomy. (b) Liver metastasis in a melanoma patient, appearing 7 years after the primary was excised.

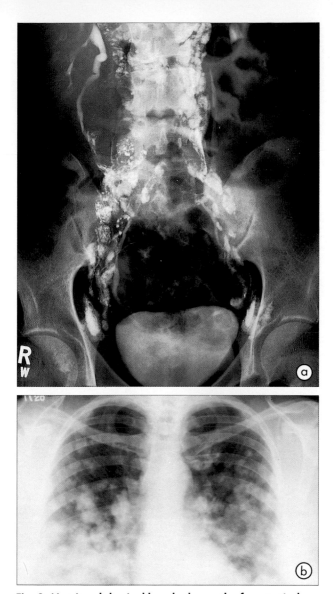

Fig. 3 Massive abdominal lymphadenopathy from testicular teratoma. It is very unusual for these tumours to metastasize widely without also involving abdominal lymph nodes. (a) This IVU lymphogram clearly shows the right ureter laterally deviated by the glandular mass. (b) Chest X-ray confirming multiple pulmonary metastases in the same patient.

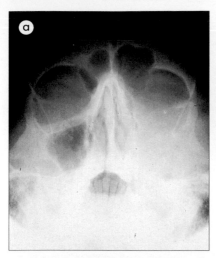

Fig. 4 Direct extension of a large maxillary carcinoma. (a) The tumour has eroded local bone structures, notably the floor of the orbit. (b) The CT confirms bone destruction in the nasal cavity and ethmoid sinus.

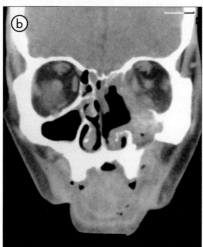

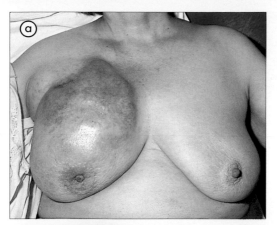

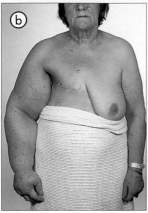

Fig. 5 Lymphatic involvement in breast cancer. (a) Axillary nodes clearly visible in a patient with a huge primary tumour occupying the whole right breast. (b) Late onset lymphadenopathy denoting local and axillary node infiltration.

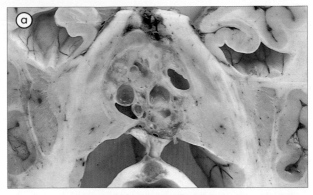

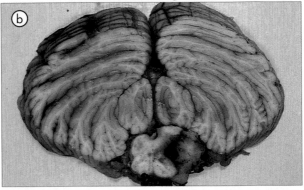

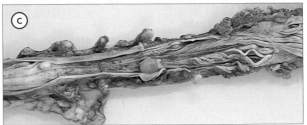

Fig. 6 Central nervous system involvement from a primary pineal teratoma. (a) Primary lesions at post-mortem. (b) Metastasis in the cerebello-pontine angle. (c) Spinal cord nodular seedlings.

Therapeutic Approaches

In order to plan the management of a particular malignant tumour the clinician needs to know:
- the histological subtype and grade;
- the apparent extent of spread of the tumour;
- the natural history of the tumour type;
- the effectiveness of available treatments.

Only when this information is available can the clinician decide whether the aim of treatment is cure or palliation. Before making a final decision the patient's general health, as well as the likely toxicity of therapy, have to be taken into account together with the wishes of the patient.

The main therapeutic options are surgery, radiotherapy, chemotherapy, and hormone therapy. The importance of simple supportive care (analgesia, antiemetics, laxatives, etc) to ameliorate symptoms — both cancer and treatment-related — should not, however be forgotten. More recently new biological therapies have been developed and some are starting to show benefit in selected tumours.

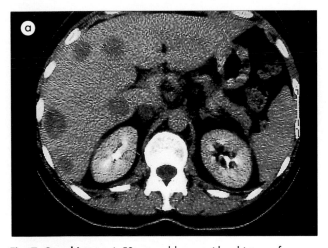

Fig. 7 Case history. A 50-year old man with a history of radical excision of a malignant melanoma of the abdominal wall, presented with back pain referred to his right leg. Investigation revealed liver (a), bone and lung metastases. He then developed an intussusception caused by tumour in the bowel. What treatment is appropriate?

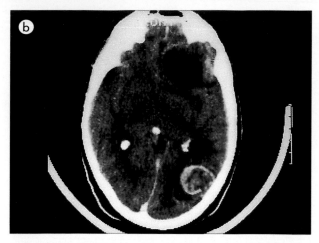

Fig. 7 contd. Case history. The patient was treated with IL-2 but the disease progressed and he developed brain metastases (b). An informed decision about therapy can only be made if both the patient and the clinician acknowledge that such treatment is entirely palliative. Only if the goals of treatment are set out from the start can unnecessary toxic treatment be avoided.

USE OF RADIOACTIVE ISOTOPES		
Isotope	Delivery	Indication
Radium-226	Intracavitary in needles	Local high doses to tumour
Iridium-192	Implanted wires	Local high dose in tumour (eg. breast, tongue)
Iodine-131	By mouth	Selective uptake by thyroid for ablation
Iodine-125	Transperineal implant	Cancer of prostate
Phosphorus-32	By IV injection	Marrow ablation
Gold-198	Intra-peritoneal colloid As gold grains	Control of ascites Intra-oral

Fig. 8 Use of radioactive isotopes.

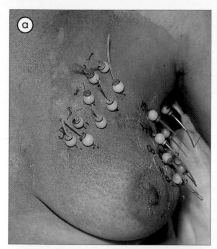

Fig. 9 Use of radioactive isotopes.
(a) Iridium-192 implant for boosting the tumour bed after excision of breast carcinoma and postoperative external radiation.
(b) X-ray confirms excellent geometry of this implant.

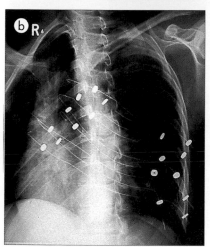

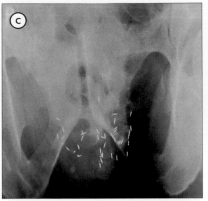

Fig. 9 contd. Use of radioactive isotopes.
(c) Transperineal iodine-125 implant for prostatic carcinoma. (d) CT scan shows seeds well positioned within the prostate. This technique has been facilitated by the advent of transrectal ultrasonography, allowing excellent imaging of this organ. In this patient with locally advanced disease, the alternative would have been a radical course of external beam radiotherapy or radical surgical excision.

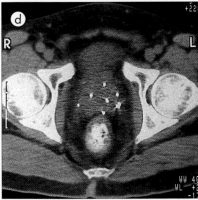

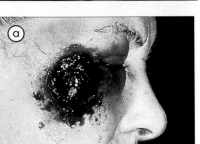

Fig. 10 Infection in neutropenic and immunosuppressed patients.
(a) Pseudomonas infection in patient with multiple myeloma.

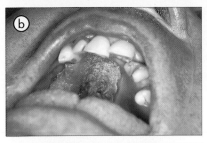

Fig. 10 contd. Infection in neutropenic and immunosuppressed patients.
(b) Fungal plaque eroding into the hard palate in a patient with leukaemia.
(c) Disseminated herpes zoster with encephalitis, pneumonitis and hepatitis. (d) The consequences of trigeminal herpes zoster infection. In this example the infection affected the ophthalmic division of the left trigeminal nerve.

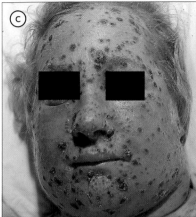

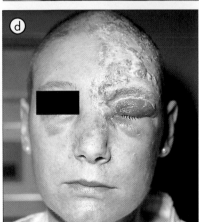

11

Investigations

A number of investigative techniques are used both to confirm the diagnosis and to assess the characteristics and degree of spread of a tumour. This latter function is referred to as staging.

Radiological techniques such as computed tomography (CT) scanning, ultrasound imaging, and magnetic resonance imaging (MRI) are widely used in the investigation of cancers.

Fig. 11 (facing) Anatomical staging of non-small cell lung cancer. In the TNM system the T stage increases with size of the tumour, its position and the degree of invasion of surrounding structures; the N stage increases as more central node areas are involved; and the M status records the presence or absence of distant metastases.

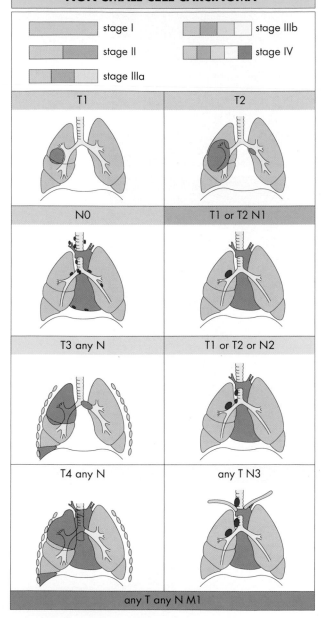

ANATOMICAL STAGING OF NON-SMALL CELL CARCINOMA

stage I
stage II
stage IIIa
stage IIIb
stage IV

| T1 | T2 |

| N0 | T1 or T2 N1 |

| T3 any N | T1 or T2 or N2 |

| T4 any N | any T N3 |

any T any N M1

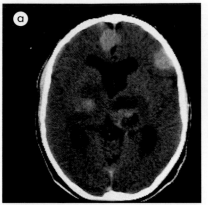

Fig. 12
Appropriate use of CT imaging.
(a) The CNS: CT image showing enhancement of multiple gliomas. (b) & (c) The head and neck: patient with an orbital lymphoma, clearly shown in CT image. Courtesy of Dr R. Blaquire.

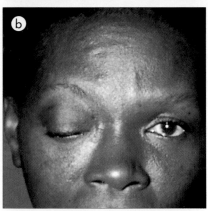

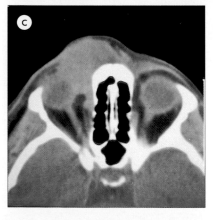

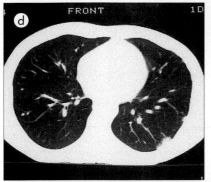

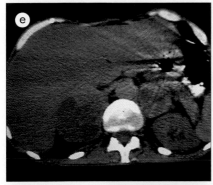

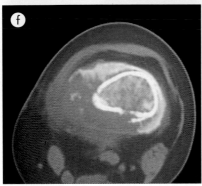

Fig. 12 contd. Appropriate use of CT imaging.
(d) The thorax: CT image showing small metastasis in the periphery of the left lung of a man treated for testicular teratoma. Different windows are used to examine the lungs and solid structures.
(e) The abdomen and pelvis: CT image showing left adrenal mass in patient with small cell lung cancer.
(f) Bone: CT image showing femoral destruction and soft tissue mass in a case of Ewing's sarcoma. Courtesy of Dr R. Blaquire.

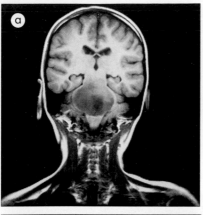

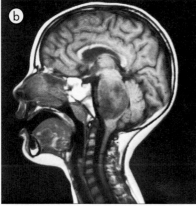

Fig. 13 MRI showing a brain stem tumour.
(a) & (b) MRI provides excellent images of the head and neck, and the CNS. As well as offering excellent resolving power, MRI scanning may be employed as a means of avoiding unpleasant invasive procedures. Spinal lesions, for example, may be adequately imaged by MRI without the need for myelography.

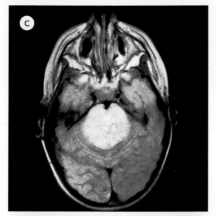

Fig. 13 contd. MRI showing a brain stem tumour. Comparison of the MRI scan (c) with the CT scan of the brain (d) shows the extra information provided by MRI.

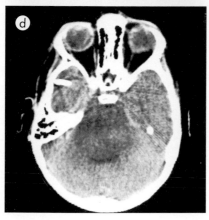

Brain Tumours

Three important groups of syndromes may occur in the presentation of brain tumours:

- 'focal neurological deficit' relating to the specific site. For example, a tumour of the dominant hemisphere, situated in the cortex close to the motor strip, may produce neurological damage resulting in hemiplegia.
- development of 'late onset epilepsy' presenting with a variety of epiletiform seizure patterns.
- symptoms resulting from 'raised intracranial pressure' (ICP), chiefly headache, nausea, visual disturbance (particularly diplopia), and drowsiness.

In addition to these major symptom clusters, pituitary tumours may cause a variety of endocrine effects as well as local structural damage from direct local extension.

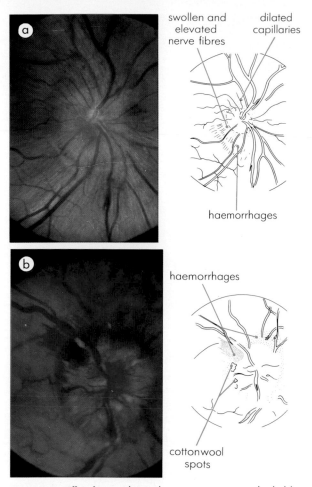

Fig. 14 Papilloedema. This is the most common and reliable physical sign of ICP. (a) Early papilloedema. Dilatation of nerve bundle fibres is clearly seen, together with superficial haemorrhages and hyperaemia of the disc margins. (b) Gross papilloedema. The disc is grossly swollen with dilated nerve fibres masking the blood vessels at the disc borders. There are haemorrhages into the nerve fibre layer around the disc, and cottonwool spots on the disc surface. Courtesy of Mr D. J. Spalton.

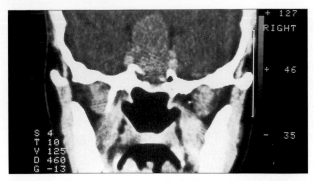

Fig. 15 Pituitary adenoma. Coronal CT scan showing large pituitary adenoma with massive suprasellar extension. The lesion, a non-functioning pituitary adenoma, presented with classic bitemporal hemianopia.

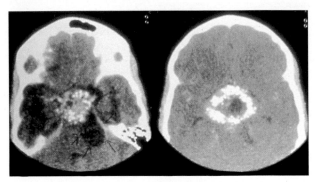

Fig. 16 Craniopharyngioma. Transaxial CT scan showing characteristic massive local calcification. For this reason, craniopharyngiomas are often not fully resectable. Courtesy of Dr H. Okazaki. By permission of Mayo Foundation.

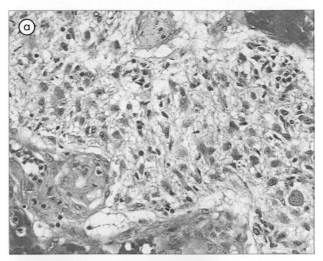

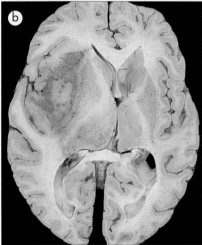

Fig. 17 High-grade astrocytoma (glioblastoma multiforme).
(a) Histologically, these tumours are characterized by increased
cellularity, pleomorphism, vascular hypertrophy and endothelial
proliferation together with areas of necrosis and haemorrhage.
(b) This glioblastoma of the left insula shows a low density
central area, with visible heterogeneity and a substantial mass
effect, displacing the anterior part of the lateral ventricle.
Courtesy of Dr H. Okazaki. By permission of Mayo Foundation.

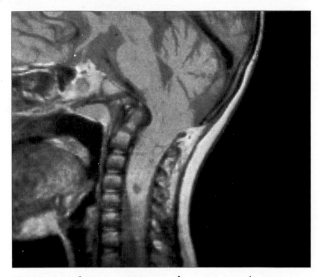

Fig. 18 Ependymoma. MRI scan of primary spinal ependymoma showing cord expansion with a small cystic component in the cervical region.

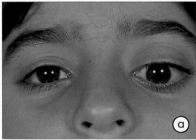

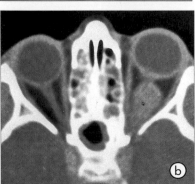

Fig. 19 Optic nerve glioma.
(a) Unilateral proptosis of the left eye, the commonest presenting feature.
(b) There was a large optic nerve glioma involving the whole of the left optic nerve.

Cancer of the Head and Neck

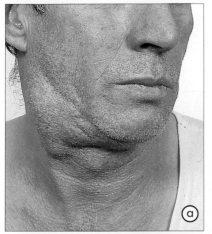

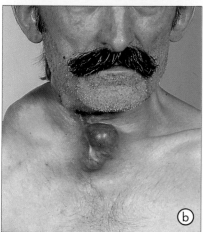

Fig. 20 Lymph node metastases. These may be the presenting feature in head and neck tumours and they are diagnostically of great importance. (a) Carcinoma of the tonsil with typical mid-cervical node. (b) Chordoma with widespread central and supraclavicular neck metastases.

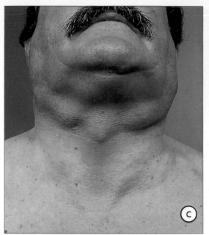

Fig. 20 contd. Lymph node metastases.
(c) Diffuse lymphoma with bilateral bulky lymphadenopathy.
(d) Anaplastic carcinoma of the thyroid with typical mass anteriorly situated in the neck and lower cervical node metastases.

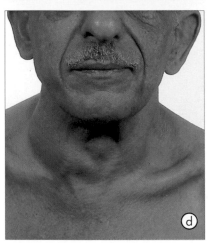

Fig. 21 (facing) The relationship of neck node involvement to primary tumour site.

THE RELATIONSHIP OF NECK NODES TO PRIMARY SITES

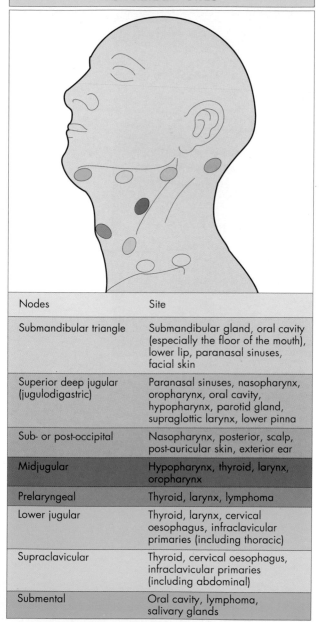

Nodes	Site
Submandibular triangle	Submandibular gland, oral cavity (especially the floor of the mouth), lower lip, paranasal sinuses, facial skin
Superior deep jugular (jugulodigastric)	Paranasal sinuses, nasopharynx, oropharynx, oral cavity, hypopharynx, parotid gland, supraglottic larynx, lower pinna
Sub- or post-occipital	Nasopharynx, posterior, scalp, post-auricular skin, exterior ear
Midjugular	Hypopharynx, thyroid, larynx, oropharynx
Prelaryngeal	Thyroid, larynx, lymphoma
Lower jugular	Thyroid, larynx, cervical oesophagus, infraclavicular primaries (including thoracic)
Supraclavicular	Thyroid, cervical oesophagus, infraclavicular primaries (including abdominal)
Submental	Oral cavity, lymphoma, salivary glands

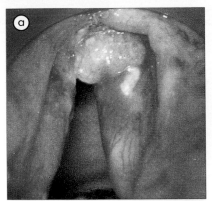

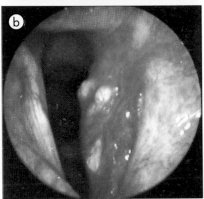

Fig. 22 Carcinoma of the vocal cords. (a) Carcinoma of the anterior vocal cords (commissure). (b) Carcinoma of the right vocal cord — direct view.

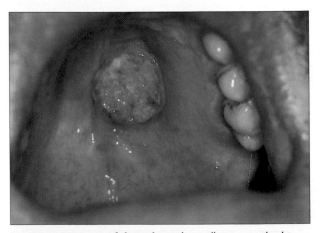

Fig. 23 Carcinoma of the palate. This well circumscribed palatal tumour was detected on a routine dental examination.

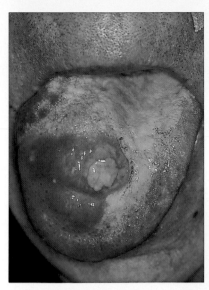

Fig. 24 Carcinoma of the tongue. This is a locally advanced tumour which has erupted through the dorsum of the tongue and was also visible on the inferior surface.

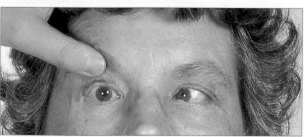

Fig. 25 Cranial nerve palsies from local extension to the base of the brain from a large carcinoma of the nasopharynx. This patient has been asked to look towards the right side. The ophthalmoplegia of the right eye is caused by a sixth nerve palsy; she also had a ptosis on the right.

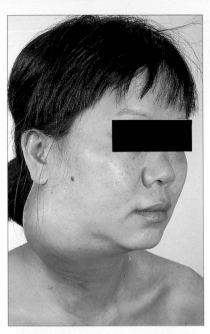

Fig. 26 Carcinoma of the nasopharynx. This patient presented with massive nodes in the right side of the neck and CT scan confirmed complete replacement of the nasopharynx and bone destruction by the primary tumour. Following radiotherapy the neck mass resolved entirely.

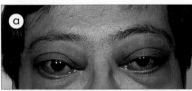

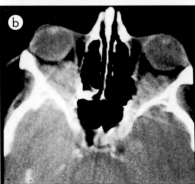

Fig. 27 Orbital pseudotumour (low-grade lymphoma). (a) Chemosis. (b) CT scan shows bilateral soft tissue swellings in the region of the posterior orbit causing bilateral proptosis and ophthalmoplegia.

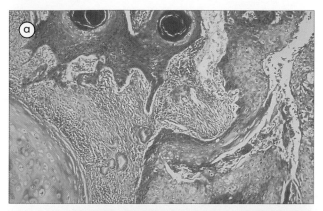

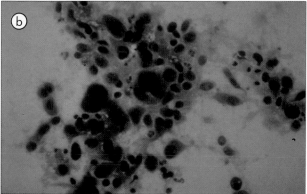

Fig. 28 Histological varieties of lung cancer. (a) Squamous cell carcinoma. Bands of tumour cells show stratification and keratinization with formation of distinctive keratin 'pearls'. (b) Large cell carcinoma (bronchial brushing, cytological preparation). The cells have clear pleomorphic nuclei that lack the denseness seen in small cell carcinoma, and a moderate amount of cytoplasm that lacks evidence of mucus storage and keratinization. Courtesy of Prof B. Corrin.

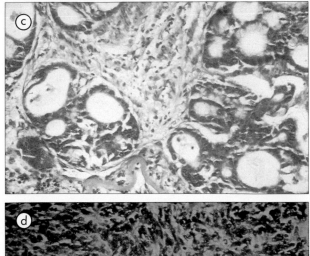

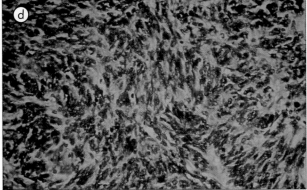

Fig. 28 contd. Histological varieties of lung cancer.
(c) Adenocarcinoma, showing prominent glandular
differentiation. (d) Small cell carcinoma consisting of spindle or
'oat' shaped cells with dense nuclei, moulded cellular
morphology and sparse cytoplasm. Courtesy of Prof B. Corrin.

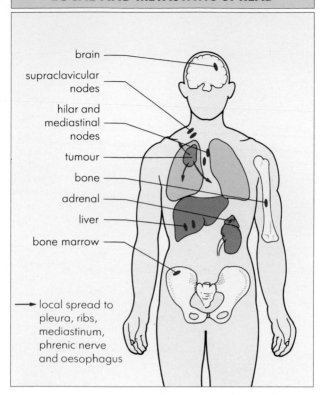

Fig. 29 Local and distant spread in small cell carcinoma of the lung.

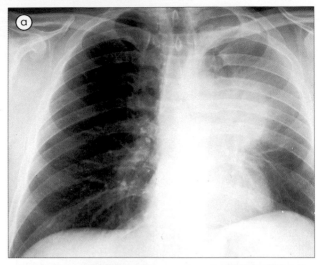

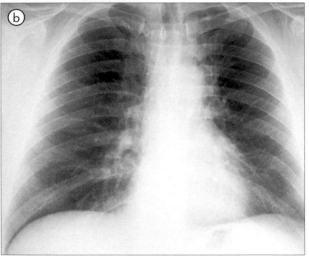

Fig. 30 Small cell carcinoma of the bronchus.
(a) Appearance before treatment. (b) Dramatic tumour
reduction following three months of combination chemotherapy.

CRITERIA FOR OPERABILITY

No obvious distant metastases

Usually only non-small cell varieties considered

General condition of the patient adequate for the planned operation

No clinically evident pleural effusion

Hilar lymphadenopathy may be acceptable, but not central mediastinal disease

Tumour >2cm from carina

Negative abdominal CT scanning

Age *per se* unimportant

Fig. 31 Criteria for operability in non-small cell lung cancer.

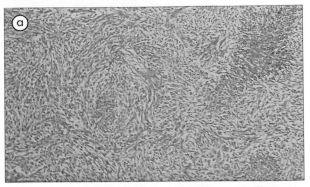

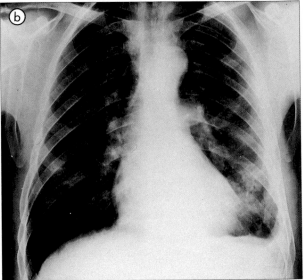

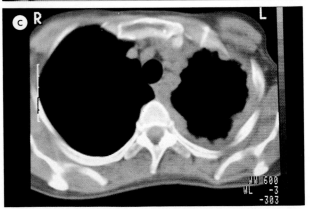

34

Fig. 32 (facing) Mesothelioma. (a) The histological appearance is variable but in this specimen the epithelial cell type adenocapillary structures are prominent, and there is an area of necrosis. Courtesy of Prof B. Corrin. (b) Typical X-ray findings, including pleural shadowing with nodulation behind the heart, in the costophrenic angle and along the lateral chest wall, together with partial destruction of ribs. Courtesy of Dr M. E. Hodson. (c) Typical CT scan appearance, with involvement of the whole of the pleura of the left lung with complete sparing on the right.

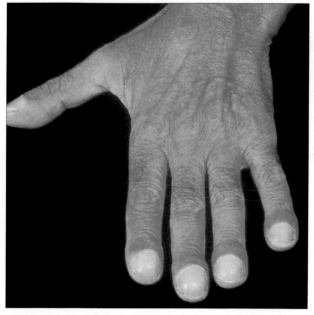

Fig. 33 Finger clubbing. This is present in about 30% of all cases of lung cancer. Courtesy of Dr M. E. Hodson.

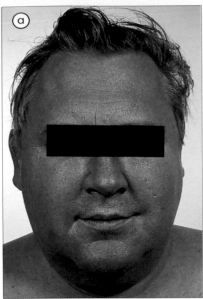

Fig. 34 Superior vena cava obstruction (SVCO). Carcinomas situated in the right main or upper lobe bronchus may cause SVCO. (a) Appearance prior to treatment, showing bloating and plethora of the face and neck. (b) Six weeks after palliative radiotherapy.

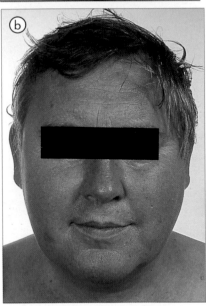

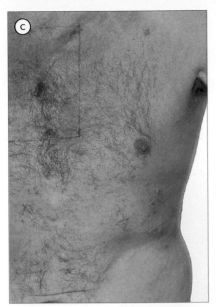

**Fig. 34 contd.
Superior vena cava
obstruction (SVCO).**
(c) Typical vascular
changes over the
chest wall, with
prominent small
purple venules.

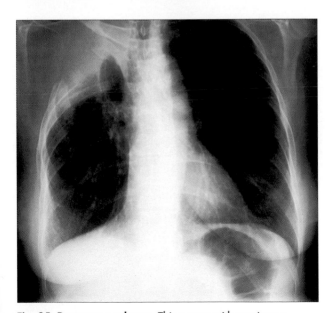

Fig. 35 Pancoast syndrome. This occurs with carcinoma
arising at the apex of the lung. There is gross destruction of the
first four ribs and upper chest wall. The pain was so severe that
this patient eventually required a cordotomy.

Breast Cancer

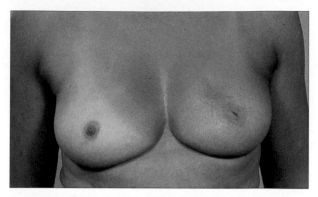

Fig. 36 Nipple inversion. An important clinical sign in breast cancer.

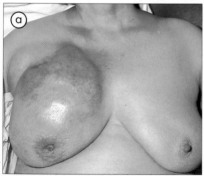

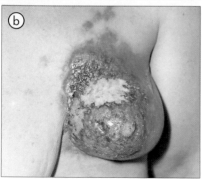

Fig. 37 Locally advanced breast cancer. (a) Massive tumour occupying most of the right breast and about to fungate. There is nipple inversion, visible axillary lymphadenopathy and *peau d'orange*. (b) Fungating tumour occupying whole breast with skin satellite nodules.

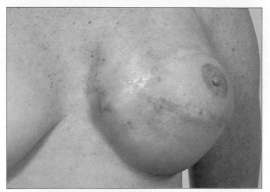

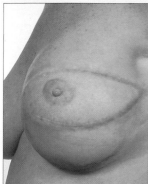

Fig. 38 Breast reconstruction with free flap grafting and modelling of nipple, taken from vulval skin.

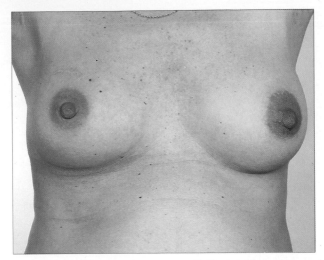

Fig. 39 Typical cosmetic appearance following lumpectomy and local irradiation for early carcinoma of the right breast. Taken approximately five years after treatment.

Gastrointestinal Cancer

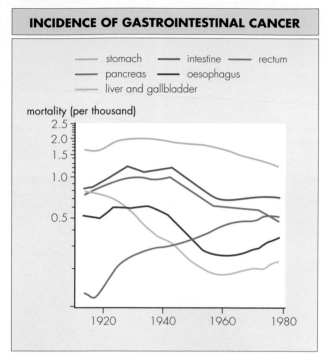

INCIDENCE OF GASTROINTESTINAL CANCER

stomach intestine rectum
pancreas oesophagus
liver and gallbladder

mortality (per thousand)

Fig. 40 Relative incidence of gastrointestinal cancer, over a sixty year period. The major changes are in the gradual decline of carcinoma of the stomach, together with an increased incidence of carcinoma of the pancreas over the same period.

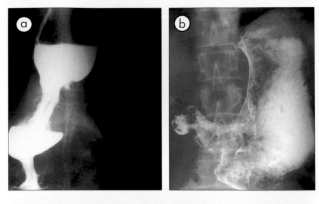

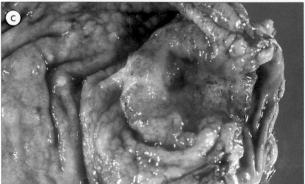

Fig. 41 Upper gastrointestinal cancer. (a) Barium swallow showing typical features of a malignant stricture of the oesophagus. There is obvious 'shouldering' of the barium column, and the length of the stricture is clearly demonstrated. (b) Large malignant gastric ulcer of the inferior prepyloric portion of the stomach. (c) This large, exophytic gastric adenocarcinoma has a central ulcerated area, which gives it a fungating appearance. Courtesy of Dr F. A. Mitros.

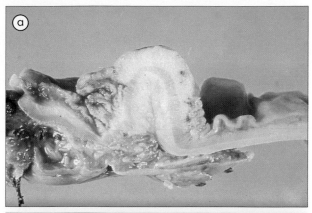

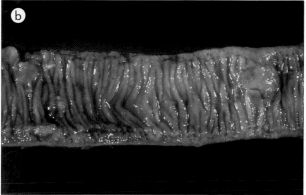

Fig. 42 Small bowel carcinoid tumour. (a) In this ileal lesion, the tumour has resulted in formation of a knuckle of bowel, with hypertrophy of the involved muscle, which is expanded by tumour, together with direct involvement of the serosa. (b) In this relatively short segment of ileum, there are four grossly identifiable carcinoids. The largest lesion, towards the right, is ulcerated, an unusual feature, and has a typical pale yellow colour. Courtesy of Dr F. A. Mitros.

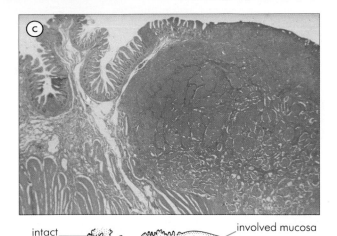

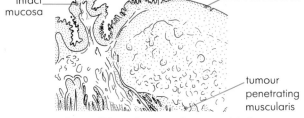

intact mucosa

involved mucosa

tumour penetrating muscularis

Fig. 42 contd. Small bowel carcinoid tumour. (c) This carcinoid of the terminal ileum is typical of an early lesion. Courtesy of Dr F. A. Mitros.

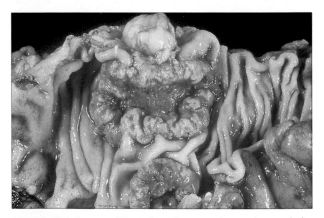

Fig. 43 Carcinoma of the colon. The central irregular eroded area and everted rolled edge are typical features. Although the tumour was relatively small, obliteration of the muscle and puckering of the wall both indicate transmural extension. Courtesy of Dr F. A. Mitros.

DISTRIBUTION OF COLORECTAL CANCER

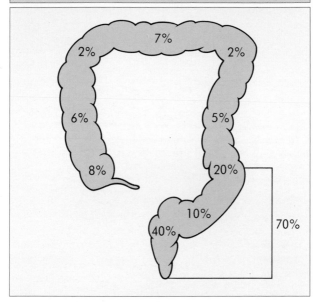

Fig. 44 Distribution of colorectal carcinoma, by large bowel site.

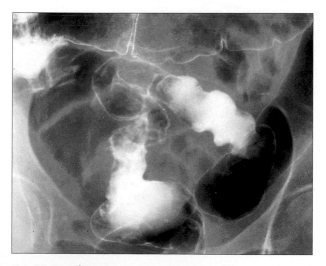

Fig. 45 Rectal carcinoma. Barium enema appearance in rectal carcinoma showing typical malignant stricture formation.

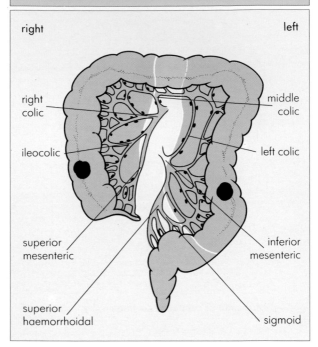

RIGHT AND LEFT HEMICOLECTOMY

right   left

right colic

middle colic

ileocolic

left colic

superior mesenteric

inferior mesenteric

superior haemorrhoidal

sigmoid

Fig. 46 Extent of resection in right and left hemicolectomy procedures for carcinomas of the colon. For tumours of the ascending colon, resection should be undertaken well beyond the hepatic flexure. For lesions of the descending colon, this part of the bowel together with the splenic flexure will need to be resected. End-to-end anastomosis can generally be performed at the primary procedure. Major arteries are indicated.

ADENOCARCINOMA OF THE PANCREAS

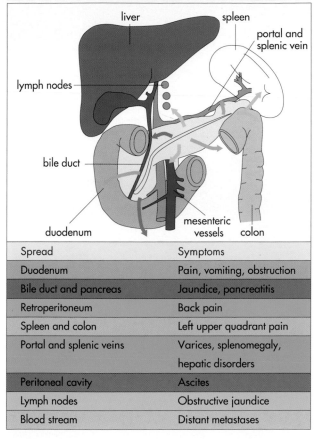

Spread	Symptoms
Duodenum	Pain, vomiting, obstruction
Bile duct and pancreas	Jaundice, pancreatitis
Retroperitoneum	Back pain
Spleen and colon	Left upper quadrant pain
Portal and splenic veins	Varices, splenomegaly, hepatic disorders
Peritoneal cavity	Ascites
Lymph nodes	Obstructive jaundice
Blood stream	Distant metastases

Fig. 47 Sites of spread and production of symptoms in adenocarcinoma of the pancreas. Courtesy of Prof. R. L. Souhami.

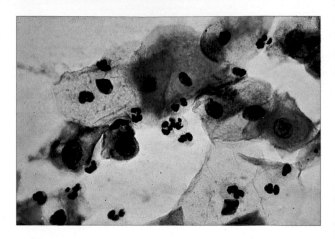

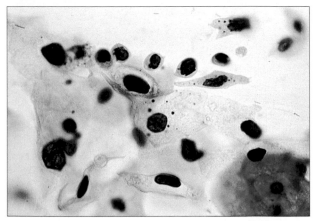

Fig. 48 Exfoliative cytology (cervical smear preparations) in carcinoma of the cervix. (a) CIN I showing mild dysplasia, dyskaryosis and slight nuclear atypia. (b) CIN II showing moderate dysplasia, with nuclear hyperchromasia and fine chromatin clumping. Courtesy of Prof C. Gompel.

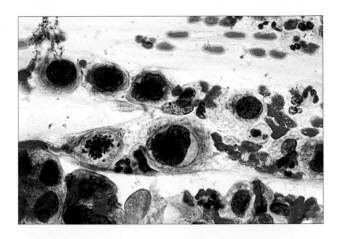

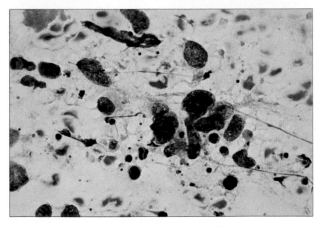

Fig. 48 contd. Exfoliative cytology (cervical smear preparations) in carcinoma of the cervix. (c) CIN II or Cis. The neoplastic cells are larger, with severe dysplasia and marked nuclear atypia. (d) Invasive squamous cell carcinoma, large cell non-keratinizing type. The cells are pleomorphic and there is a necrotic background. Courtesy of Prof C. Gompel.

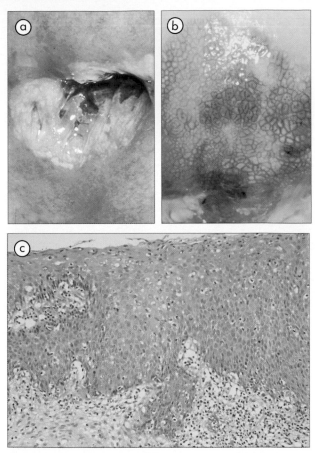

Fig. 49 Colposcopic views of the cervix. (a) and (b) Aceto white staining and typical mosaic pattern of pre-invasive carcinoma. Colposcopic techniques give far greater detail than is possible by conventional out-patient examination. Courtesy of Mr A. C. Silverstone. (c) Colposcopic biopsy showing micro-invasive carcinoma in a field of CIN III. No tumour was visible to the naked eye.

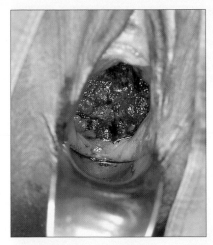

Fig. 50 Typical appearance of locally advanced carcinoma of the cervix at examination under anaesthesia. In this case the cervix was almost totally destroyed, and there was obvious involvement of the vaginal fornices.

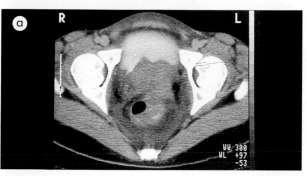

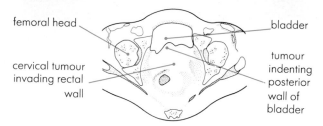

Fig. 51 CT scanning in carcinoma of the cervix. (a) Large central tumour with obvious extension posteriorly to the rectal wall, and indenting the bladder anteriorly.

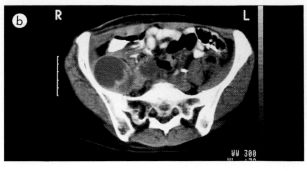

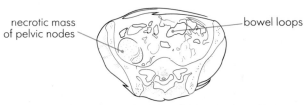

necrotic mass
of pelvic nodes

bowel loops

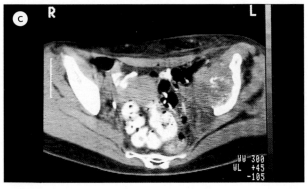

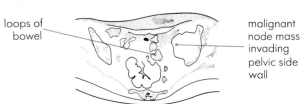

loops of
bowel

malignant
node mass
invading
pelvic side
wall

Fig. 51 contd. CT scanning in carcinoma of the cervix.
(b) Large necrotic mass of iliac nodes adjacent to pelvic side
wall. (c) Local pelvic erosion from large mass of left sided pelvic
nodes.

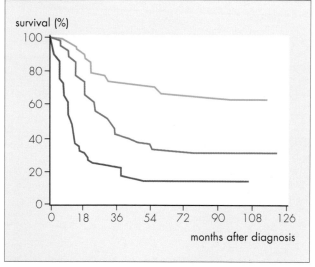

SURVIVAL IN INVASIVE CARCINOMA OF THE CERVIX

Risk group	No. of patients	No. of deaths	Median DFST (months)
—Good (IIa⁻, IIb⁻)	66	22	92+
—Intermediate (IIb⁺, IIIa⁻, IIIb⁻)	62	34	31
—Poor (IIIa⁺, IIIb⁺)	50	35	11

Fig. 52 Disease-free survival time (DFST) following treatment of invasive carcinoma of the cervix. FIGO staging gives excellent prognostic information, with wide variation in survival largely dependent on tumour stage. Superscripts indicate lymph node status, based on lymphogram findings. [Data from Hammond, J. A. *et al.* (1981) *Int. J. Rad. Oncol. Biol. Phys.* **7**, 1713–1718.]

TYPICAL SYMPTOMS OF OVARIAN CARCINOMA	
Pelvic and/or abdominal mass	95%
Non-specific abdominal discomfort	75%
Abdominal bloating	55%
Early satiety	45%
Ascites	40%
Masses in pouch of Douglas	40%
Weight loss	30%
Shortness of breath	20%
Vaginal bleeding	10%
Urinary frequency	10%
Pleural effusion	10%

Fig. 53 Symptoms and signs of ovarian cancer.

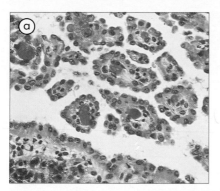

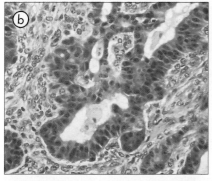

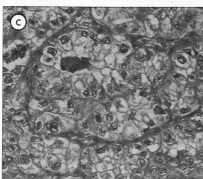

Fig. 54 Histological subtypes in ovarian carcinoma. (a) Papillary ovarian carcinoma, well differentiated, showing early invasive features. (b) Ovarian carcinoma with endometrioid features. The glands are not well formed in all areas, and are losing their differentiation. (c) Clear-cell carcinoma showing typical features and a glandular pattern.

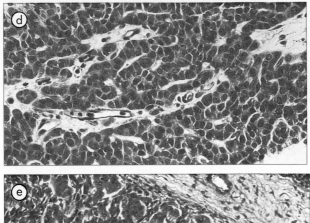

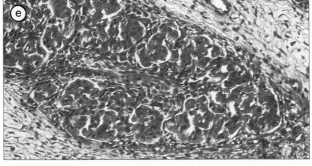

Fig. 55 Histological subtypes in ovarian carcinoma.
(d) Granulosa cell carcinoma, with epithelial cells in nests
containing small follicular spaces, with solid cords of darkly
staining cells. (e) Sertoli–Leydig cell tumour showing nests of
epithelial cells forming rudimentary tubules, a potentially
malignant tumour of moderate differentiation. Courtesy of Prof
J. D. Woodruff.

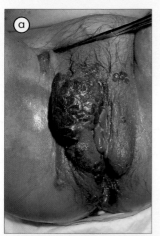

Fig. 56 Carcinoma of the vulva. (a) This was a particularly advanced case presenting as a rapidly expanding mass on the anterior part of the right labium majora. The patient then rapidly developed skin satellite nodules, and ipsilateral inguinal nodes. (b) CT scan confirmed massive extension upwards to the perirectal fascia and the rectum itself.

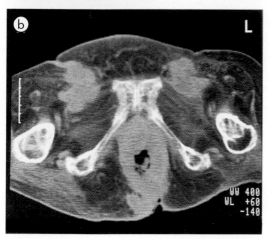

DEPTH OF INVASION AND STAGING IN BLADDER CANCER

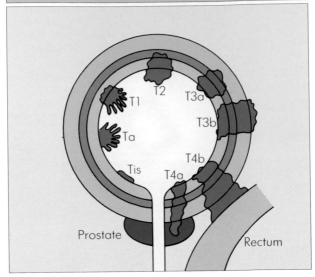

Fig. 57 Staging of bladder cancer. Relationship between depth of invasion and T stage for bladder cancer.

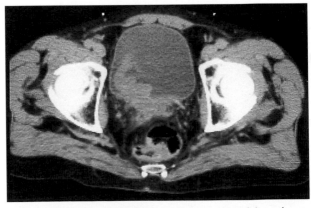

Fig. 58 CT imaging in bladder cancer. CT scan of the pelvis showing extensive tumour within the bladder and posteriorly on the rectum. Courtesy of Dr R. Blaquire.

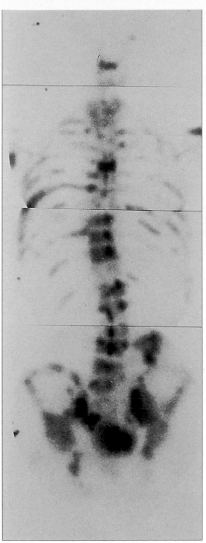

Fig. 59 Bone imaging in prostate cancer. Image shows extensive bony involvement of the spine and pelvis prior to treatment.

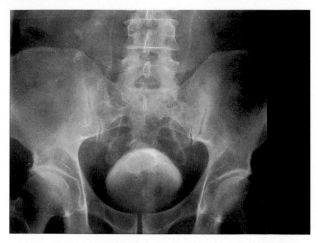

Fig. 60 Prostatic carcinoma. IVU showing gross prostatic hypertrophy elevating the bladder and indenting the bladder base. This apparently benign lesion contained adenocarcinoma.

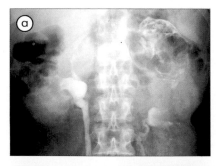

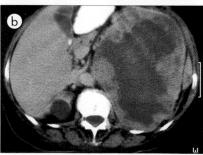

Fig. 61 Calcified renal cancer and tumour imaging. (a) IVU showing a grossly calcified renal cell carcinoma of the upper pole of the left kidney. The calyceal pattern on that side is distorted. (b) CT image of the abdomen showing a massive left renal cell carcinoma filling most of the left side of the abdomen. The renal vein remains patent. Courtesy of Dr R. Blaquire.

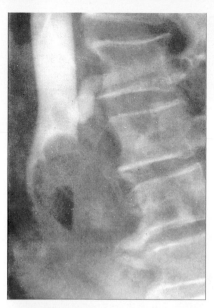

Fig. 62 Renal cell carcinoma. Venogram showing extensive tumour thrombus occluding the inferior vena cava.

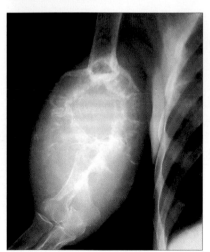

Fig. 63 Gross destructive bone metastasis from renal cell carcinoma.

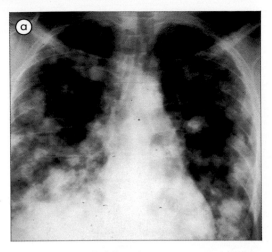

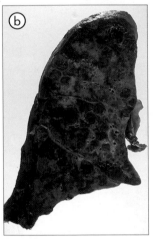

Fig. 64 Lung metastasis from testicular cancer. (a) Diffuse lung involvement by metastatic choriocarcinoma of the testis. The patient presented with dyspnoea and haemoptysis and was unaware of a testicular mass (see also Fig. 3). Courtesy of Dr G. Mead. (b) Post mortem appearance of the lung of a patient with extensive choriocarcinoma of the testis. The patient died shortly after the first cycle of chemotherapy — all the lung nodules sampled showed necrosis without viable malignant teratoma. Courtesy of Dr J. Theaker.

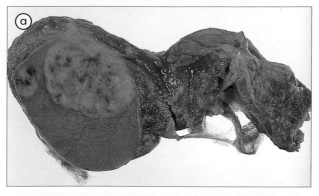

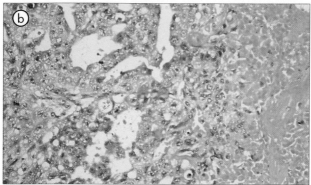

Fig. 65 Macroscopic and microscopic appearance of testicular teratoma. (a) Macroscopic appearance showing two nodules of teratoma within the testis. (b) Microscopic appearance of typical malignant teratoma intermediate. Courtesy of Dr J. Theaker.

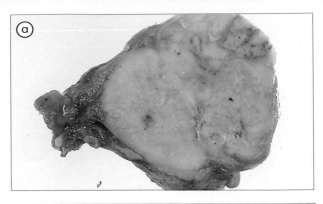

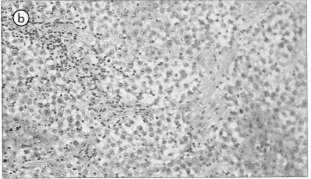

Fig. 66 Macroscopic and microscopic appearance of testicular seminoma. (a) Macroscopically there are small areas of necrosis which are commonly seen in large seminomas. (b) Classic microscopic appearance of seminoma.

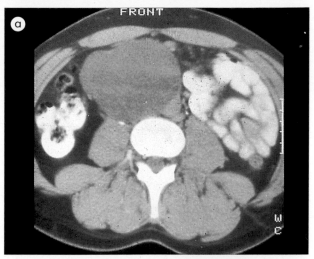

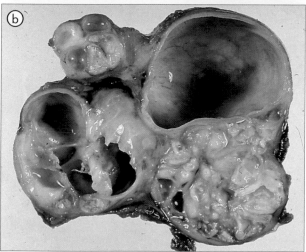

Fig. 67 Resected residual teratoma. (a) CT image of an extensive residual mass after chemotherapy for testicular teratoma. (b) Surgical specimen of resected mass — teratoma differentiated. Left *in situ* such benign tumours may continue to grow or may transform into malignant phenotypes — carcinoma and/or sarcoma. Courtesy of Dr G. Mead.

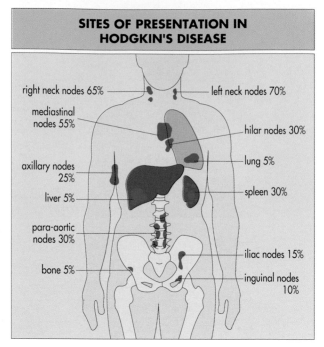

SITES OF PRESENTATION IN HODGKIN'S DISEASE

right neck nodes 65%

left neck nodes 70%

mediastinal nodes 55%

hilar nodes 30%

axillary nodes 25%

lung 5%

liver 5%

spleen 30%

para-aortic nodes 30%

iliac nodes 15%

bone 5%

inguinal nodes 10%

Fig. 68 Common sites of presentation of Hodgkin's disease.

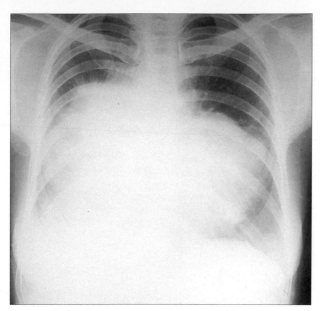

Fig. 69 Massive mediastinal involvement in Hodgkin's disease. Tracheal or bronchial compression may occur even when mediastinal involvement is much less obvious.

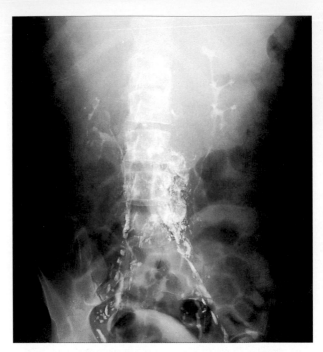

Fig. 70 Lymphangiography and IVU showing enlarged foamy para-aortic lymph nodes involved with Hodgkin's disease. The left kidney is displaced laterally by a mass of unfilled involved lymph nodes. CT imaging provides information on upper abdominal nodes, mesenteric nodes and organs, whilst lymphangiography provides detailed information on the size and architecture of para-aortic and pelvic lymph nodes.

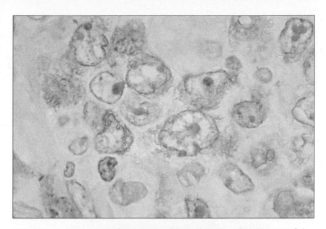

Fig. 71 Immunocytochemistry of lymphoma. The nature of the tumour can be confirmed by use of monoclonal antibodies directed against epitopes in specific tissues. In this case the tumour is common leucocyte antigen positive and antibodies for lambda are also positive with brown peroxidase pigment. Kappa staining was negative confirming that this is a monoclonal lambda B cell neoplasm.

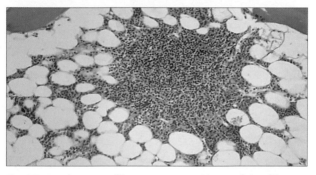

Fig. 72 Involvement of bone marrow with a nodule of low-grade lymphoma.

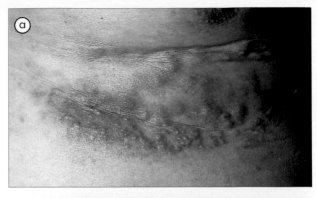

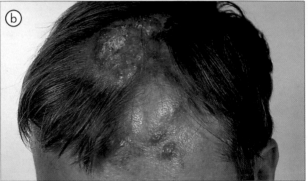

Fig. 73 Skin involvement in non-Hodgkin's lymphoma.
(a) Nodular skin recurrence of high-grade lymphoma. (b) Gross
exophytic recurrence of high-grade lymphoma on the scalp.

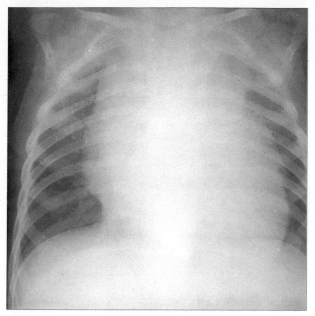

Fig. 74 T-cell lymphoblastic leukaemia. There is a typical large mediastinal mass in this one-year-old old with lymphoblastic leukaemia. Courtesy of Dr A. Smith.

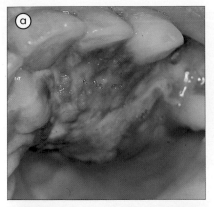

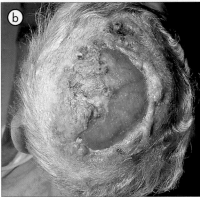

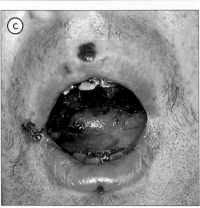

Fig. 75 Infection in acute myelogenous leukaemia (AML) induction. In addition to bacterial infection, fungal, viral and opportunistic infections are common. (a) Severe oral candidiasis in AML. Courtesy of Dr A. Smith. (b) Pyoderma gangrenosum. Bacterial infections may be severe and unusual in their behaviour. (c) Severe oral mucositis due to neutropenia. Such mucosal damage provides an easy portal of entry for pathogenic organisms. Courtesy of Prof J. Whitehouse.

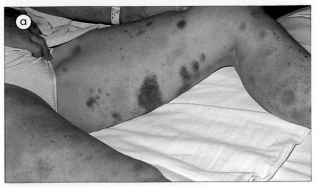

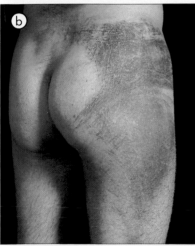

Fig. 76
Consequences of thrombocytopenia.
(a) Multiple bruises on the legs of a patient with AML.
(b) Intramuscular injection should always be avoided in the presence of thrombocytopenia. This picture illustrates the consequences of a single 1ml injection.
(c) Antibiotic rash with purpura in a patient with AML.

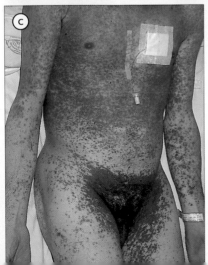

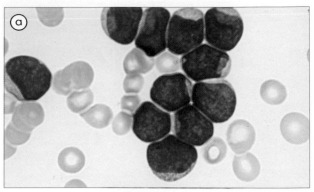

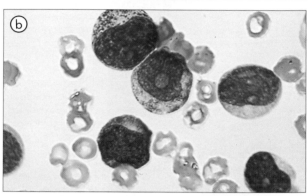

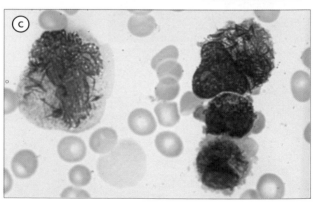

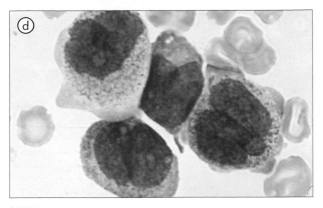

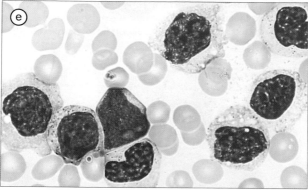

Fig. 77 Classification of acute myelogenous leukaemia.
(a) M₁ subtype. Blast cells have large irregular nuclei with one
or more nucleoli. The cytoplasm is often placed eccentrically.
Auer rods are uncommon. (b) M₂ subtype. Blast cells are often
folded with several nucleoli and azurophilic granules and
occasional Auer rods. (c) M₃ subtype. Promyelocytes contain
coarse azurophilic granules and so called 'faggots' or Sultan
bodies made up of aggregates of granules. (d) M₃ subtype
(microgranular type). These promyelocytes contain many small
azurophilic granules. (e) M₄ subtype (myelomonocytic
leukaemia) showing blasts with cytoplasmic granules (myelo- and
promyeloblasts) together with blasts with cytoplasmic vacuoles
and folded nuclei (microblasts). Courtesy of Prof A. V.
Hoffbrand.

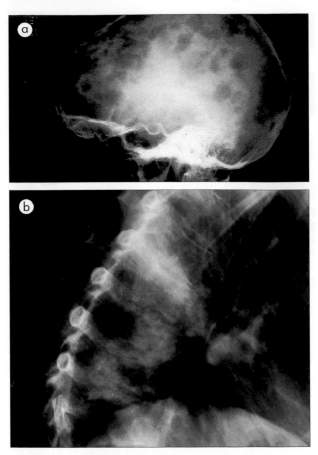

Fig. 79 Lytic bone lesions. This is an important diagnostic finding in multiple myeloma. (a) Radiograph of multiple lytic lesions of the skull. (b) Radiograph of the spine showing typical severe demineralization with vertebral collapse.

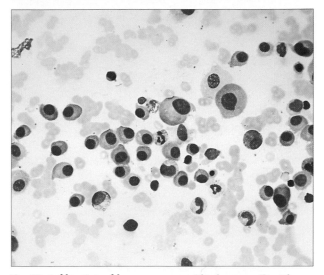

Fig. 80 Infiltration of bone marrow with plasma cells. Often regarded as the key diagnostic feature of multiple myeloma.

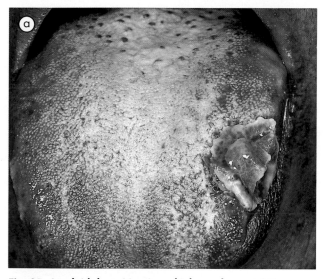

Fig. 81 Amyloid deposition in multiple myeloma. (a) Tongue infiltrated with amyloid showing macroglossia and ulceration. The waxy appearance is typical of amyloid deposition. Courtesy of Prof A. V. Hoffbrand.

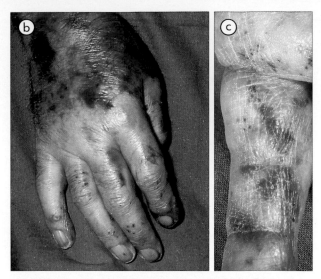

Fig. 81 contd. Amyloid deposition in multiple myeloma.
(b) Amyloid infiltration of skin of the hands. The skin is waxy
and there is purpura (c). Courtesy of Prof A. V. Hoffbrand.

Skin Cancer

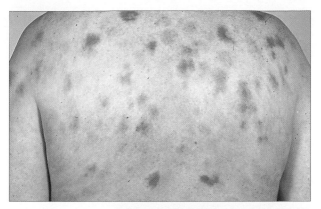

Fig. 82 Mycosis fungoides. One of several types of skin lymphoma. There is often an erythematous or pre-tumour stage, but this patient exhibits the classical features of infiltrative or plaque-type disease. Later these lesions often enlarge and ulcerate; internal organ involvement may occur.

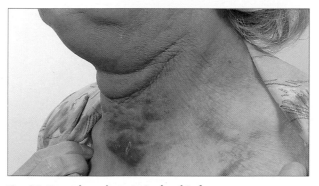

Fig. 83 Secondary deposits in the skin from a squamous carcinoma of the bronchus. This patient had a number of nodules in the anterior part of the neck which eventually coalesced.

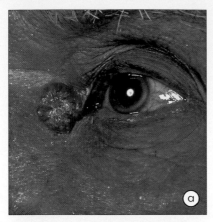

Fig. 84 Basal cell carcinomas. (a) A typical lesion situated at the inner canthus with clearly defined margins and a typical pearly edge. Courtesy of Dr A. du Vivier. (b) Ulcerating basal cell carcinoma situated beneath the left columella.

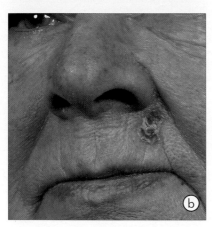

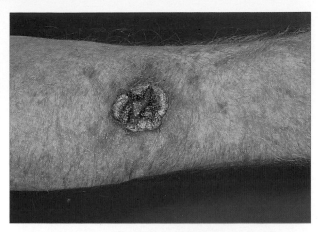

Fig. 85 Squamous cell carcinoma of the forearm. In this site, squamous carcinomas are more common than basal carcinomas, through the appearance in this case is similar to that of a rodent ulcer. This tumour required surgical excision.

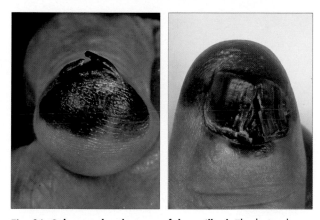

Fig. 86 Subungual melanoma of the nailbed. The lesion has an irregular outline and its colours vary from black to grey and blue. As it invades, the lesion distorts and splits the nailplate. Such lesions are not usually so grossly abnormal. Courtesy of Dr A. C. Pembroke.

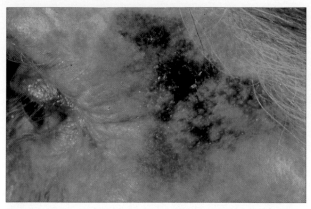

Fig. 87 Lentigo maligna. Here occurring in a typical site as a flat, irregular, slowly-enlarging tumour. Courtesy of Dr A. du Vivier.

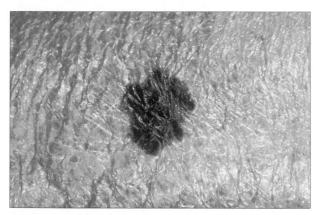

Fig. 88 Superficial spreading melanoma. A more sharply demarcated lesion. Courtesy of Dr A. du Vivier.

Bone and Soft Tissue Sarcoma

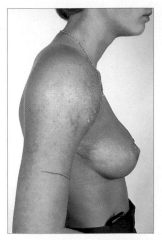

Fig. 89 Osteosarcoma. Typical clinical features, showing a firm smooth swelling at the site of the tumour (see also Fig. 90 (b)).

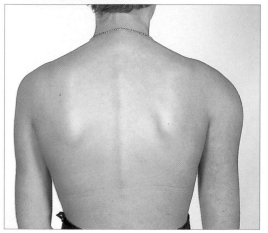

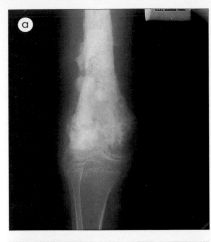

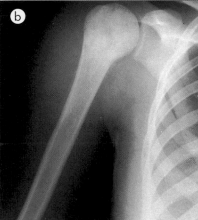

Fig. 90 Radiological features of osteosarcoma. (a) Osteosarcoma of lower tibia showing massive new bone formation together with destructive change and soft tissue swelling. (b) Osteosarcoma of upper humerus showing major soft tissue involvement, periosteal elevation of the lateral aspect, and new bone formation of the upper humerus (same case as in Fig. 89).

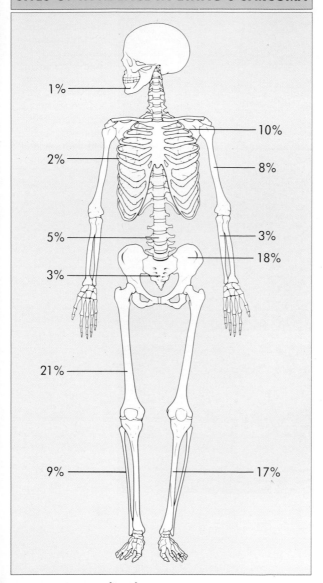

Fig. 91 Main sites of incidence in Ewing's sarcoma.

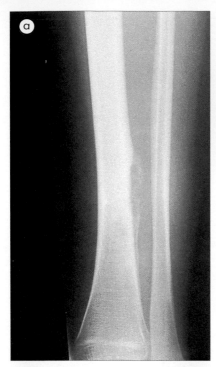

Fig. 92 Ewing's sarcoma. (a) In this lesion of the lower tibia, there is major periosteal elevation and 'saucerization' of the affected bone. (b) Ewing's sarcoma of the right ileum, with bone expansion and destruction of the acetabulum.

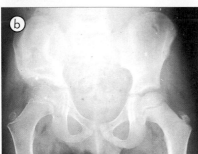

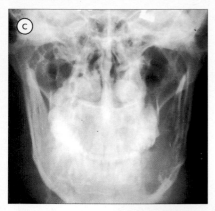

Fig. 92 contd. Ewing's sarcoma. (c) Left mandible with massive destruction of the whole of the upper table and normal appearances on the right side.

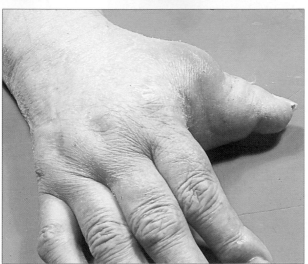

Fig. 93 Chondrosarcoma of the base of the thumb. Typically, this was an elderly patient with a three year history of a slowly enlarging mass.

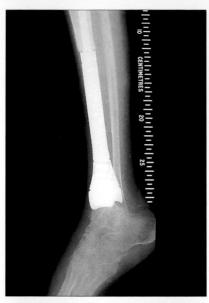

Fig. 94 Prosthetic replacement of lower tibia in Ewing's sarcoma. (Same case as in Fig. 92(a)).

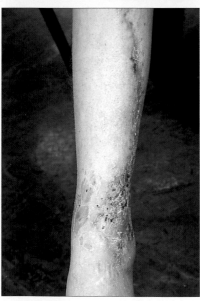

Childhood Tumours

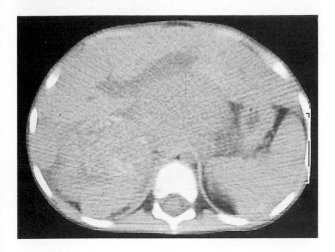

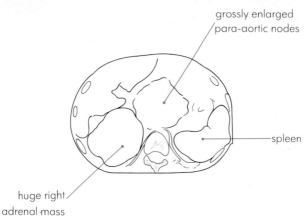

grossly enlarged
para-aortic nodes

spleen

huge right
adrenal mass

Fig. 95 Neuroblastoma presenting as an adrenal mass. CT
scan showing a large right adrenal mass with calcification and
grossly enlarged para-aortic lymph nodes.

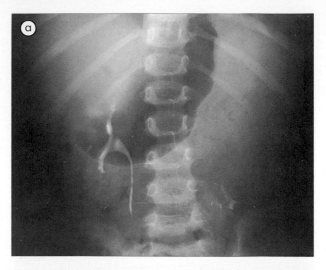

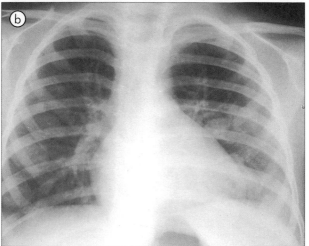

Fig. 96 Wilms' tumour. (a) IVU showing a large left-sided Wilms' tumour pushing the stomach to the right, depressing the kidney and distorting the renal pelvis. (b) Chest X-ray showing numerous pulmonary metastases, each measuring several centimetres in diameter.

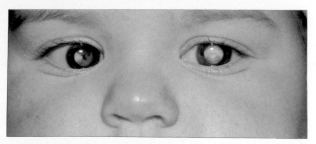

Fig. 97 Retinoblastoma. Bilateral leucocoria with gross ocular involvement. Courtesy of Mr D. J. Spalton.

Supportive and Terminal Care

The symptomatic care of cancer patients is of paramount importance at all stages of the disease. In addition to specific treatment of symptoms, it should not be forgotten that emotional and practical support are often as important, and sometimes more important, than pharmaceutical intervention.

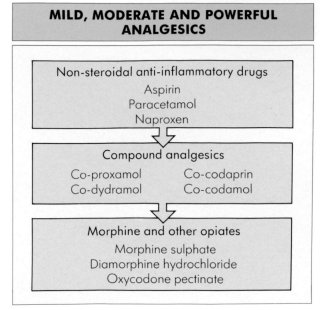

MILD, MODERATE AND POWERFUL ANALGESICS

Non-steroidal anti-inflammatory drugs
Aspirin
Paracetamol
Naproxen

Compound analgesics
Co-proxamol   Co-codaprin
Co-dydramol   Co-codamol

Morphine and other opiates
Morphine sulphate
Diamorphine hydrochloride
Oxycodone pectinate

Fig. 98 Mild, moderate and powerful analgesics. Patients should be maintained on mild analgesics until the maximum recommended dose fails to control pain. They are then moved onto a moderate analgesic, until once again the maximum recommended dose fails. They then progress to a powerful analgesic.

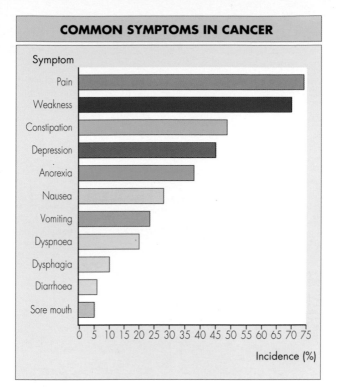

COMMON SYMPTOMS IN CANCER

Symptom

Pain
Weakness
Constipation
Depression
Anorexia
Nausea
Vomiting
Dyspnoea
Dysphagia
Diarrhoea
Sore mouth

0 5 10 15 20 25 30 35 40 45 50 55 60 65 70 75

Incidence (%)

Fig. 99 Common symptoms in 100 consecutive patients with a variety of different cancers. The majority of these problems can be efficiently and rapidly dealt with by intelligent use of the appropriate supportive measures. Dyspnoea is probably the most difficult and resistant symptom to control effectively, but pain, nausea and constipation usually respond well to modern pharmacological therapy.

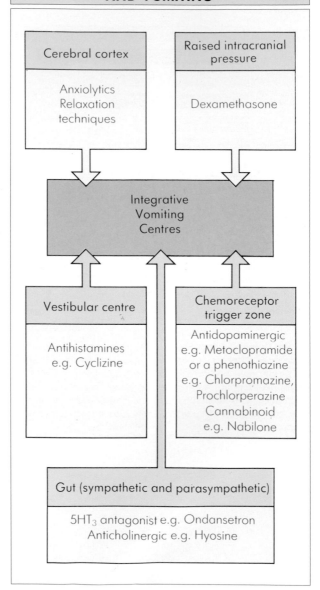

Fig. 100 Mechanisms of nausea and vomiting and effective drugs.

Index